Slow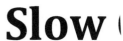

Enjoy Delicious Dishes While Losing Weight And Quickly

Burning Fat

(Slow Cooker Recipes For Beginners)

Perry Shaw

Table Of Contents

Chicken Bowl

Ingredients:

- 2 teaspoon fresh onion powder
- 2 cup tomatoes, chopped
- 2 cup of water
- 2 teaspoon olive oil
- 2 -pound chicken breast, skinless, boneless, chopped
- 2 cup sweet corn, frozen
- 2 teaspoon ground paprika

Directions

1. Mix chopped chicken breast with ground paprika and fresh onion powder.
2. Transfer it to the slow cooker.

3. Add water and sweet corn. Cook the mixture on High for 4 hours.

4. Then drain the liquid and transfer the mixture to the bowl.

5. Add tomatoes and olive oil. Mix the meal.

Asian Style Chicken

Ingredients:

- 2 oz. scallions, chopped
- 1 cup of orange juice
- 2 teaspoon ground coriander
- 2 pound chicken breast, skinless, boneless, roughly chopped
- 2 teaspoon hot sauce
- 1/2 cup of soy sauce
- 2 teaspoon sesame oil

Directions

1. Put all ingredients in the slow cooker.
2. Close the lid and cook the meal on Low for 8-8 ½ hours.

3. Then transfer the chicken and a little amount of the chicken liquid to the bowls.

Oregano Chicken Breast

Ingredients:

- 2 bay leaf
- 2 teaspoon peppercorns
- 2 teaspoon salt
- 2 cups of water
- 2 -pound chicken breast, skinless, boneless, roughly chopped
- 2 tablespoon dried oregano

Directions

1. Pour water into the slow cooker and add peppercorns and bay leaf.

2. Then sprinkle the chicken with the dried oregano and transfer it to the slow cooker.

3. Close the lid and cook the meal on High for 4 hours.

Thai Chicken

Ingredients:

- 2 teaspoon chili powder
- 2 teaspoon tomato paste
- 2 teaspoon ground cardamom
- 2 cup of water
- 4 oz. chicken fillet, sliced
- 1 cup of coconut milk
- 2 teaspoon dried fresh lemon grass

Directions

1. Rub the chicken with chili powder, tomato paste, ground cardamom, and dried fresh lemon grass. Transfer it to the slow cooker.

2. Add water and coconut milk.

3. Close the lid and cook the meal on High for 4 hours.

Chicken Teriyaki

Ingredients:

- 2 carrot, chopped
- 2 onion, chopped
- 2 teaspoon butter
- 2 -pound chicken wings
- 1 cup teriyaki sauce
- 1 cup of water

Directions

1. Toss butter in the pan and melt it.

2. Add fresh onion and carrot and roast the vegetables for 10 minutes over medium heat.

3. Then transfer them to the slow cooker.

4. Add chicken wings, teriyaki sauce, and water.

5. Close the lid and cook the meal for 4 hours on High.

Stuffed Chicken Breast

Ingredients:

- 2 teaspoon olive oil
- 2 teaspoon salt
- 2 cup of water
- 2 -pound chicken breast, skinless, boneless
- 2 tomato, sliced
- 2 oz. mozzarella, sliced
- 2 teaspoon fresh basil

Directions

1. Make the horizontal cut in the chicken breast in the shape of the pocket.

2. Then fill it with sliced mozzarella, tomato, and basil.

3. Secure the cut with the help of the toothpicks and sprinkle the chicken with olive oil and salt.

4. Place it in the slow cooker and add water.

5. Cook the chicken on low for 6 hours.

Chicken Pate

Ingredients:

- 2 -pound chicken liver
- 2 cups of water
- 2 tablespoons coconut oil
- 2 carrot, peeled
- 2 teaspoon salt

Directions

1. Chop the carrot roughly and put it in the slow cooker.

2. Add chicken liver and water.

3. Cook the mixture for 8 hours on Low.

4. Then drain water and transfer the mixture to the blender.

5. Add coconut oil and salt.

6. Blend the mixture until smooth.

7. Store the pate in the fridge for up to 8 days.

   Nutrition: calories 2 10 0, fat 10 , carbs 2, protein 2 8

Chicken Masala

Ingredients:

- 2 cup of coconut milk
- 2 -pound chicken fillet, sliced
- 2 teaspoon olive oil
- 2 teaspoon gram masala
- 2 teaspoon ground ginger

Directions

1. Mix coconut milk with ground ginger, gram masala, and olive oil.

2. Add chicken fillet and mix the ingredients.

3. Then transfer them to the slow cooker and cook on High for 4 hours.

Chicken Minestrone

Ingredients:

- 2 teaspoon ground paprika
- 2 teaspoon ground cumin
- 2 cup Swiss chard, chopped
- 1/2 cup red kidney beans, canned
- 35 oz. chicken fillet, sliced
- 2 cup of water
- 2 cup tomatoes, chopped
- 2 teaspoon chili powder

Directions
1. Sprinkle the chicken fillet with chili powder, ground paprika, and ground cumin.

2. Transfer it to the slow cooker.

3. Add tomatoes, water, Swiss chard, and red kidney beans.

4. Close the lid and cook the meal on High for 4-4 ½ hours.

French-Style Chicken

Ingredients:

- 1 cup celery stalk, chopped
- 2 teaspoon dried tarragon
- 1/2 cup white wine
- 2 can fresh onion soup
- 4 chicken drumsticks

Directions

1. Put ingredients in the slow cooker and carefully mix them.

2. Then close the lid and cook the chicken on low for 8 hours.

Sweet Chicken Breast

Ingredients:

- 1 cup of water
- 2 -pound chicken breast, skinless, boneless
- 2 teaspoon curry paste
- 2 red onions
- 2 tablespoons of liquid honey
- 2 tablespoon butter

Directions

1. Rub the chicken breast with curry paste and transfer it to the slow cooker.

2. Slice the fresh onion and add it to the cooker too.

3. Then add water and close the lid.

4. Cook the chicken breast on High for 4 hours.

5. After this, toss the butter in the skillet.

6. Melt it and add chicken.

7. Sprinkle the chicken with liquid honey and roast for 2 minute per side.

8. Slice the chicken breast.

Basil Chicken

Ingredients:

- 2 teaspoon dried oregano

- 2 -pound chicken fillet, sliced

- 2 teaspoon mustard

- 2 tablespoons balsamic vinegar

- 2 cup of water
- 2 teaspoon dried basil

Directions

1. Mix chicken fillet with mustard and balsamic vinegar.

2. Add dried basil, oregano, and transfer to the slow cooker.

3. Add water and close the lid.

4. Cook the chicken on low for 8 hours.

Bbq Chicken

Ingredients:

- 2 tablespoon avocado oil
- 4 tablespoons fresh lemon juice
- 1 cup of water
- 8 oz. chicken fillet, sliced

- 2 teaspoon minced garlic
- 1 cup BBQ sauce

Directions

1. Put in the bowl BBQ sauce, minced garlic, avocado oil, and fresh lemon juice.
2. Add chicken fillet and mix the mixture.
3. After this, transfer it to the slow cooker. Add water and close the lid.
4. Cook the chicken on low for 8 hours.

Sugar Chicken

Ingredients:

- 2 tablespoon fresh lemon juice

- 2 teaspoon ground black pepper

- 1/2 cup milk

- 2 teaspoon chili flakes

- 6 chicken drumsticks

- 2 tablespoons brown sugar

- 2 tablespoon butter, melted

Directions

1. In the bowl, mix chili flakes, brown sugar, butter, fresh lemon juice, and ground black pepper.

2. Then brush every chicken drumstick with the sweet mixture and transfer it to the slow cooker.

3. Add milk and close the lid. Cook the meal on Low for 6 hours.

Chicken And Peppers

Ingredients:

- 1 teaspoon rosemary, dried
- 1 teaspoon coriander, ground
- 2 teaspoon Italian seasoning
- A pinch of cayenne pepper
- 2 cup chicken stock
- 2   pound chicken breasts, skinless, boneless, and cubed
- 1/2 cup tomato sauce
- 2 red bell peppers, cut into strips
- 2 teaspoon olive oil

Directions:

1. In your Slow Cooker, mix the chicken with the peppers, tomato sauce, and the other ingredients, toss, put the lid on and cook on Low for 6 hours.

2. Divide everything between plates and serve.

Chicken Chowder

Ingredients:

- 2 teaspoon garlic powder
- 4 bacon strips, cooked and crumbled
- A pinch of salt and black pepper
- 2 tablespoon parsley, chopped
- 4 chicken breasts, skinless and boneless and cubed

- 4 cups chicken stock

- 2 sweet potato, cubed

- 8 ounces canned green chilies, chopped

- 2 yellow onion, chopped

- 35 ounces coconut cream

Directions:

1. In your Slow Cooker, mix chicken with stock, sweet potato, green chilies, onion, garlic powder, salt and pepper, stir, cover, and cook on Low for 6 hours and 45 minutes.

2. Add coconut cream and parsley, stir, cover, and cook on Low for 10 minutes more.

3. Ladle chowder into bowls, sprinkle bacon on top, and serve.

Parsley Turkey Breast

Ingredients:

- 2 teaspoon fresh onion powder
- 2 teaspoon garlic powder
- 2 teaspoon parsley flakes
- 2 teaspoon thyme, dried
- 2 teaspoon sage, dried
- 2 teaspoon paprika, dried
- 4 pounds turkey breast, bone in
- 2 cup black figs
- 4 sweet potatoes, cut into wedges
- 1 cup dried cherries, pitted
- 2 white onions, cut into wedges
- 1 cup dried cranberries
- 1/2 cup water

- A pinch of sea salt

- Black pepper to the taste

Directions:

1. Put the turkey breast in your Slow Cooker, add sweet potatoes, figs, cherries, onions, cranberries, water, parsley, garlic and fresh onion powder, thyme, sage, paprika, salt and pepper, toss, cover and cook on Low for 8 hours.

Chili Chicken

Ingredients:
- 2 teaspoon garlic, minced

- 1 cup of water

- 2 -pound chicken wings

- 2 teaspoon chili powder

- 2 tablespoon hot sauce

- 2 tablespoon coconut oil, melted

- 1 teaspoon ground turmeric

Directions

1. Rub the chicken wings with hot sauce, chili powder, ground turmeric, garlic, and coconut oil.

2. Then pour water into the slow cooker and add prepared chicken wings.

3. Cook the chicken on low for 8 hours.

Orange Chicken

Ingredients:

- 2 teaspoon olive oil

- 2 teaspoon salt

- 2 cup of water

- 2 -pound chicken breast, skinless, boneless, sliced

- 2 orange, chopped

- 2 teaspoon ground turmeric

- 2 teaspoon peppercorn

Directions

1. Put all ingredients in the slow cooker and gently mix them.

2. Close the lid and cook the meal on Low for 8 hours.

3. When the time is finished, transfer the chicken to the serving bowls and top with orange liquid from the slow cooker.

Bacon Chicken

Ingredients:

- 1 cup of water
- 1/2 tomato juice
- 2 teaspoon salt
- 1 teaspoon ground black pepper
- 4 bacon slices, cooked
- 4 chicken drumsticks

Directions

1. Sprinkle the chicken drumsticks with salt and ground black pepper.

2. Then wrap every chicken drumstick in the bacon and arrange it in the slow cooker.

3. Add water and tomato juice.

4. Cook the meal on Low for 8 hours.

Bourbon Chicken Cubes

Ingredient

- 2 white onion, diced
- 2 teaspoon garlic powder
- 2 -pound chicken fillet, cubed
- 1 cup bourbon
- 2 teaspoon liquid honey
- 2 tablespoon BBQ sauce

Directions

1. Put all ingredients in the slow cooker.

2. Mix the mixture until liquid honey is dissolved.

3. Then close the lid and cook the meal on high for 4 hours.

Mexican Chicken

Ingredients:

- 2 red onion, sliced
- 1 cup salsa Verde
- 2 cup of water
- Sweet pepper, sliced
- Cayenne pepper

Directions

1. Pour water into the slow cooker.

2. Add salsa Verde and onion.

3. Then add cayenne pepper and chicken thighs.

4. Cook the mixture on High for 4 hours.

5. After this, add sweet pepper and cook the meal on Low for 4 hours.

Curry Chicken Wings

Ingredients:

- 1 cup heavy cream
- 2 teaspoon minced garlic
- 1 teaspoon ground nutmeg
- 1 cup of water
- 2 -pound chicken wings

- 2 teaspoon curry paste

Directions

1. In the bowl, mix curry paste, heavy cream, minced garlic, and ground nutmeg.

2. Add chicken wings and stir.

3. Then pour water into the slow cooker.

4. Add chicken wings with all remaining curry paste mixture and close the lid.

5. Cook the chicken wings on Low for 8 hours.

Thyme Whole Chicken

Ingredients:

- 2 tablespoon olive oil

- 2 teaspoon salt

- 2 cup of water

- 4 -pound whole chicken

- 2 tablespoon dried thyme

Directions

1. Chop the whole chicken roughly and sprinkle with dried thyme, olive oil, and salt.

2. Then transfer it to the slow cooker, add water.

3. Cook the chicken on low for 10 hours.

Fennel And Chicken Sauté

Ingredients:

- 2 cup of water

- 2 teaspoon ground black pepper

- 2 teaspoon olive oil

- 1 teaspoon fennel seeds

- 2 cup fennel, peeled, chopped

- 35 oz. chicken fillet, chopped

- 2 tablespoon tomato paste

Directions
1. Heat the olive oil in the skillet.

2. Add fennel seeds and roast them until you get a saturated fennel smell.

3. Transfer the seeds to the slow cooker.

4. Add fennel, chicken fillet, tomato paste, water, and ground black pepper.

5. Close the lid and cook the meal on Low for 8 hours.

   Nutrition: calories 2 00, fat 10 , carbs 4 , protein 8

Russian Chicken

Ingredients:

- 2 teaspoon ground black pepper
- 2 teaspoon sunflower oil
- 2 teaspoon salt
- 1 cup of water
- 2 tablespoons mayonnaise
- 4 chicken thighs, skinless, boneless
- 2 teaspoon minced garlic

Directions

1. In the bowl, mix mayonnaise, minced garlic, ground black pepper, salt, and oil.

2. Then add chicken thighs and mix the ingredients well.

3. After this, pour water into the slow cooker. Add chicken thighs mixture.

4. Cook the meal on High for 4 hours.

Creamy Sea Bass

Ingredients:

- 2 -pound sea bass fillets, boneless
- 2 teaspoon garlic powder
- 1 teaspoon Italian seasoning
- 1 teaspoon salt
- 1/2 cup heavy cream
- 2 tablespoon butter

Directions:

1. In the slow cooker, mix the sea bass with the other ingredients.

2. Close the slow cooker lid and cook for 2 hours on High.

Oregano Crab

Ingredients:

- ¾ teaspoon minced garlic
- 2 tablespoon fresh lemon juice
- 1 cup of coconut milk
- 2 tablespoon dried oregano
- 2 cups crab meat
- 1 cup spring onions, chopped

Directions:

1. In the slow cooker, mix the crab with oregano and the other ingredients and close the lid

2. Cook for 45 minutes on High, divide into bowls, and serve.

Parmesan Salmon

Ingredients:

- 4 oz Parmesan, grated
- 2 tablespoons lime juice
- 2 teaspoon minced garlic
- 1/2 cup fresh chives, chopped
- 8 oz salmon fillets, boneless
- 2 teaspoon cayenne pepper
- 2 teaspoon chili pepper
- 1 cup coconut cream

Directions:

1. In the slow cooker, mix the salmon with the coconut cream and the other ingredients and close the lid.

2. Cook on High for 2-2 ½ hours and45 minutes and serve.

Balsamic Mussels

Ingredients:

- 2 teaspoon fresh lemon juice
- 2 tablespoon sesame oil
- 1/2 cup butter
- 4 tablespoons coconut cream
- 2 -pound mussels
- 2 tablespoon Balsamic vinegar
- 1 teaspoon stevia extract
- 2 teaspoon fresh lemon zest

Directions:

1. In the slow cooker, mix the mussels with vinegar, stevia, and the other ingredients.

2. Close the slow cooker lid and cook the catfish for 2 hours on High.

3. Divide into bowls and serve.

Spicy Tuna

Ingredients:

- 1 teaspoon salt
- 2 jalapeno pepper, chopped
- 1/2 cup coconut oil
- 2 garlic clove, chopped
- 4 oz tuna fillet
- 2 tablespoon olive oil
- 2 teaspoon hot paprika
- 2 red chili pepper minced
- 1 teaspoon black pepper

Directions:

1. Put the oil in the slow cooker.

2. Add the fish and the other ingredients and toss gently.

3. Close the lid and cook the oil mixture on High for 2 hour.

4. Divide between plates and serve.

   Nutrition: calories 4 010 , fat 2 2, carbs 2 , protein 2 10

Turmeric Calamari

Ingredients:

- 1 teaspoon minced garlic
- 2 tablespoon heavy cream
- 1 teaspoon ground coriander
- 1 teaspoon salt
- 1 teaspoon black pepper
- 2 -pound calamari rings
- 2 teaspoon turmeric
- 2 teaspoon hot paprika
- 2 tablespoons coconut cream

Directions:

1. In the slow cooker, mix the calamari with the turmeric and the other ingredients and close the lid.

2. Cook the seafood for 6 hours on Low.

3. When the time is over, stir the mix and serve.

Thyme Sea Bass

Ingredients:

- 1 teaspoon dried thyme

- 2 teaspoon olive oil

- 1/2 cup water

- 2 teaspoon apple cider vinegar

- 1 teaspoon salt

- 4 oz sea bass, trimmed

- 2 tablespoons coconut cream

- 4 oz spring onions, chopped

- 2 teaspoon fennel seeds

Directions:

1. In the slow cooker, mix the sea bass with the cream and the other ingredients.

2. Close the lid and cook sea bass for 4 hours on Low.

Shrimp And Zucchini

Ingredients:

- 2 tablespoon butter, melted
- 2 teaspoon salt
- 2 tablespoon keto tomato sauce
- ¾ cup of water
- 2 -pound shrimp, peeled and deveined
- 2 zucchinis, roughly cubed
- 2 cup cherry tomatoes, halved
- 1 cup Mozzarella cheese, shredded

- 4 tablespoons cream cheese

Directions:

1. In the slow cooker, mix the shrimp with zucchinis and the other ingredients except for the cheese and toss.

2. Sprinkle the cheese on top, close the lid and cook on High for 2 hours.

Fresh Lemon Cod

Ingredients:

- 2 tablespoon chives, chopped

- 2 teaspoon turmeric powder

- 1 teaspoon salt

- 1 teaspoon ground black pepper

- 2 teaspoon butter

- 1/2 cup organic almond milk

- 25 oz cod fillet

- Juice of 2 fresh lemon

- Zest of 2 fresh lemon , grated

- 2 oz Parmesan, grated

Directions:

1. In the slow cooker, mix the cod with fresh lemon juice, zest, and the other ingredients.

2. Close the lid and cook the sauce for 2 hours on High.

3. Divide between plates and serve.

Cinnamon Mackerel

Ingredients:

- 1 teaspoon salt
- 1 teaspoon basil, dried
- 2 teaspoon cumin, ground
- ¾ teaspoon ground cinnamon
- 4 pound mackerel, trimmed
- 2 tablespoon avocado oil
- 2 teaspoon garlic powder
- 1/2 cup coconut milk

Directions:

1. In the slow cooker, mix the mackerel with the oil and the other ingredients and close the lid.

2. Cook the fish for 4-4 ½ hours on High.

3. Divide between plates and serve.

Parsley Salmon

Ingredients:

- 1 teaspoon chili flakes
- 2 teaspoon turmeric powder
- 2 oz Parmesan, grated
- 4 tablespoons coconut oil
- 35 oz salmon fillet
- 2 tablespoons parsley, chopped
- 1 cup coconut cream
- 1 teaspoon salt

Directions:

1. In the slow cooker, mix the salmon with the parsley and the other ingredients.

2. Close the lid and cook the meal for 2 hours on High.

Cheesy Tuna

Ingredients:

- 35 ounces tuna fillet, boneless and cubed
- 2 teaspoon olive oil
- 2 garlic clove, crushed
- 2 teaspoon fennel seeds
- 1 cup Cheddar, shredded
- 2 cup coconut cream
- 2 tablespoon Ricotta cheese
- 2 teaspoon salt
- 1 teaspoon white pepper

Directions:

1. In the slow cooker, mix the tuna with the cream and the other ingredients.

2. Close the lid and cook snapper for 10 hours on Low.

    Nutrition: calories 24 , fat 4.4 , fiber 4 .4 , carbs 8 .8, protein 22

Spiced Shrimp

Preparation Time: 35 minutes
Cooking time: 2 hour
Servings: 2

Ingredients:
- 2 tablespoon olive oil
- 2 tablespoon coconut cream
- 1 teaspoon salt
- 2 tablespoons water
- 8 oz shrimp, peeled and deveined

- 2 teaspoon chili powder

- 2 teaspoon nutmeg, ground

- 2 teaspoon coriander, ground

- 1 teaspoon minced garlic

Directions:

1. In the slow cooker, mix the shrimp with chili powder, nutmeg, and the other ingredients.

2. Close the lid.

3. Cook for 2 hour on High.

Seafood Stew

Ingredients:

- 2 garlic clove, diced

- ¾ teaspoon chili flakes

- 1/2 teaspoon ground black pepper

- 1/2 cup crushed tomatoes

- 1 teaspoon dried thyme

- 2 tablespoons olive oil

- 2 cup mussels

- 2 cup salmon fillet, boneless and cubed

- 2 cup shrimp, peeled and deveined

- 4 spring onions, chopped

- 1 green bell pepper, chopped

Directions:

1. In the slow cooker, mix the mussels with the salmon and the other ingredients.

2. Stir the mixture and close the lid.

3. Cook the meal for 8 hours on Low.

4. Divide into bowls and serve.

Shrimp And Green Beans

Ingredients:

- 2 teaspoon coriander, ground
- 2 teaspoon basil, dried
- ¾ cup crushed tomatoes
- 2 tablespoon olive oil
- 4 spring onions, chopped
- 2 green bell pepper, chopped
- 2 cup of water
- 2 -pound shrimp, peeled and deveined
- 1/2 pound green beans, trimmed and halved
- 2 teaspoon salt
- 2 teaspoon chili flakes

- 2 teaspoon paprika
- 1 teaspoon garam masala

Directions:

1. In the slow cooker, mix the shrimp with green beans, salt, and the other ingredients.

2. Close the lid and cook for 4 hours on High.

3. Divide into bowls and serve.

Salmon And Spinach Bake

Ingredients:

- ¾ cup organic coconut milk
- 2 teaspoon butter
- 1 teaspoon ground thyme

- 1 teaspoon salt

- 1/2 cup of water

- 2 -pound salmon fillet, chopped

- 1/2 cup spinach, chopped

- 1 cup Cheddar cheese, shredded

Directions:

1. In the slow cooker, mix the salmon with spinach and the other ingredients, toss, and close the lid.

2. Cook the salmon bake for 6-6 ½ hours on Low.

Chili Squid

Ingredients:

- 1 teaspoon chili powder

- 1 teaspoon hot paprika

- 2 tablespoon butter

- 1/2 cup heavy cream

- 2 teaspoon ground black pepper

- 2 tablespoon dried dill

- 35 oz squid tubes, trimmed

- 2 cup spring onions, chopped

- 2 teaspoon salt

Directions:

1. In the slow cooker, mix the squid with spring onions and the other ingredients.

2. Close the slow cooker lid and cook for 2.6 hours on High.

Calamari Rings And Broccoli

Ingredients:

- 4 -pound calamari rings

- 2 cup broccoli florets

- 2 jalapeno pepper, minced

- 2 tablespoon keto tomato sauce

- 1/2 cup heavy cream

- 1 teaspoon salt

- 1 teaspoon chili powder

- 2 teaspoon cumin, ground

- 2 garlic cloves, diced

- 2 tablespoon butter

Directions:

1. In the slow cooker, mix the calamari with broccoli and the other ingredients, toss and close the lid.

2. Cook the meal on Low for 4.6 hours.

Coconut Sausage Mix

Ingredients:

- 2 egg, whisked
- 1 cup Parmesan, grated
- 1/2 teaspoon ground black pepper
- 2 tablespoon fresh parsley, chopped
- 6 oz sausages, chopped
- 1 cup coconut cream
- 2 teaspoon turmeric powder
- 1 teaspoon cayenne pepper

Directions:

1. In the slow cooker, mix the sausages with the cream and the other ingredients and toss.
2. Close the lid.
3. Cook casserole for 4 hours on High.

Ricotta Frittata

Ingredients:

- 4 garlic cloves, minced
- 2 tablespoons of parsley, chopped
- Salt and black pepper- to taste
- Cooking spray
- 4 eggs, whisked
- 2 tablespoons of chives, diced
- 6 tablespoon of ricotta cheese
- 1 cup of parmesan, grated

Directions:

1. Start by greasing the base of your Crockpot.
2. Spread the peppers at the base of the pot.
3. Whisk the egg with remaining Ingredients: and pour into crockpot.

4. Cover your crockpot and select the Low settings for 6 hours.
5. Remove the crockpot's lid.
6. Slice and serve warm.

Breakfast Bowl

Ingredients:

- 2 teaspoon chili flakes
- 2 teaspoon ground black pepper
- ¾ teaspoon salt
- 2 tablespoon full-fat cream cheese
- 8 oz chicken fillets, chopped
- 2 tablespoon butter
- 4 eggs, beaten

Directions:

1. Place the butter and chicken fillets in the slow cooker.
2. Sprinkle the chicken with the chili flakes, ground black pepper, and salt.
3. Whisk the beaten fresh eggs and with the full-fat cream cheese.

4. Stir the mixture and pour it over the chicken. Mix well.
5. Close the lid and cook the breakfast for 4 hours on High.
6. Stir the cooked meal one more time and then transfer to serving bowls.
7. Enjoy!

Tapioca Chocolate Pudding

Ingredients:

- 1/2 cup of sugar-free chocolate chips
- ⅔ cup of tapioca pearls
- 8 oz. water

Directions:

1. Start by throwing all the pudding Ingredients: into the Crockpot.
2. Cover your crockpot and select the Low settings for 2 hours.
3. Remove the crockpot's lid.
4. Serve fresh.

Egg, Kale, And Mozzarella Casserole

Ingredients:

- 1/2 cup green onions, sliced
- 8 eggs, beaten
- Salt and pepper to taste
- 2 teaspoons olive oil
- 4 cup mozzarella cheese, grated

Directions:

1. Mix all ingredients in a bowl and stir to combine all ingredients.
2. Place in a Ziploc bag and write the date when the recipe is made.
3. Place inside the freezer.
4. Once you are ready to cook the meal, allow to thaw on the countertop for at least 2 hours.

5. Place in the crockpot.
6. Close the lid and cook on low for 4 hours or on high for 2 hours.

Egg And Cottage Cheese Savory Breakfast Muffins

Ingredients:

- 1/2 teaspoon gluten free baking powder
- 1/9 teaspoon salt or to taste
- Wet Ingredients:
- 4 eggs, beaten
- 2 green onion, thinly sliced
- 1/2 cup low fat cottage cheese
- 1/2 cup almond meal
- 1/2 cup parmesan cheese, finely grated
- 2 tablespoons nutritional yeast flakes
- 1/2 teaspoon spike seasoning (optional)
- 1/2 cup raw hemp seeds
- 2 tablespoons flaxseed meal

Directions:

1. Add all the dry ingredients into a bowl and mix until well combined.
2. Add all the wet ingredients into a large bowl and whisk well.
3. Add the dry ingredients into the bowl of wet ingredients, a little at a time and whisk each time.
4. When all the dry ingredients are added, spoon into greased muffin molds. Fill up to ¾ the mold.
5. Place crumpled aluminum foil at the bottom of the cooker (this step can be avoided if your cooking pot is ceramic).
6. Place the muffin molds inside the cooker.
7. Close the lid.
8. Set cooker on 'High' option and timer for 2-4 hours.

9. Check after 2 hours of cooking. If it is not looking done, then cook for some more time.

10.   If you like the top to be dry, then uncover and cook during the last 40-60 minutes of cooking.

11.   For medium top, you can place a chopstick on the top of the cooker before closing the lid.

12.   Let it cool in the cooker for a while.

13.   Cool slightly. Run a knife around the edges. Invert on to a plate and serve immediately.

Broccoli And Sausage Casserole

Ingredients:

- 6 ounces Jones Dairy farm little links (breakfast sausage) cooked, sliced
- 6 fresh eggs
- 2 clove garlic, minced
- Cooking spray
- 1 cup cheddar cheese, shredded
- 6 tablespoons whipping cream
- 1/2 teaspoon salt or to taste
- Pepper to taste

Directions:

1. Spray the inside for the slow cooker with cooking spray. Be generous with the spray.
2. Spread the broccoli at the bottom of the pot. Layer with sausage slices all over the broccoli followed by cheese.
3. Whisk together in a bowl, eggs, whipping cream, pepper, salt and garlic. Pour into the slow cooker.
4. Close the lid. Select 'Low' option and timer for 4-6 hours or on 'High' option and timer for 2-4 hours or until the edges are brown and it is not jiggling in the center.
5. Serve hot or warm.

Egg Casserole With Italian Cheeses, Sun-Dried Tomatoes And Herbs

Ingredients:

- 2 tablespoons basil, chopped
- 2 tablespoon thyme leaves
- Salt and pepper to taste
- 2 cup mixed Italian cheeses, grated
- 2 tablespoons milk
- 4 tablespoons sun-dried tomatoes, chopped
- 2 tablespoons onion, minced

Directions:
1. Mix all ingredients in a bowl.
2. Place in a Ziploc bag and write the date when the recipe is made.

3. Place inside the freezer.
4. Once you are ready to cook the meal, allow to thaw on the countertop for at least 2 hours.
5. Place all ingredients in the crockpot.
6. Cook on high for 2 hours or on low for 4 hours.

Coconut Chip Rice Pudding

Ingredients:

- 1 cup of maple syrup
- 1/2 cup of raisins
- 1/2 cup of almonds
- A pinch Cinnamon powders
- 1 cup of coconut chips
- 2 cup of almond milk
- 2 cups of water

Directions:

1. Start by throwing all the Ingredients: into the Crockpot.
2. Cover your crockpot and select the Low settings for 4 /2 hours.
3. Remove the crockpot's lid.
4. Serve fresh.

Cheesy Bacon Ham Steaks & Mushrooms

Ingredients:

- 2 shallot, thickly chopped
- 2 garlic clove, minced
- 2 tbsp. of butter
- 1 cup fresh sliced mushrooms
- 4 bacon strips, cut and lightly browned
- 2 cup shredded smoked Gouda cheese

Directions:

1. Sauté the mushrooms and shallots in a frying pan with the butter for a couple of minutes.
2. Season with salt and pepper to taste and add the garlic last.
3. Place the ham leg pieces onto the slow cooker and pour the mushrooms on top.

4. Set and cook on low heat for 4 hours.
5. Add the cheese during the last 25 minutes of cooking.
6. Serve.

Avocado Tuna Balls

Ingredients:

- 6 oz tuna
- 2 egg
- 2 teaspoon olive oil
- 2 tablespoon coconut flakes, unsweetened
- 2 avocado, pitted, peeled
- 2 tablespoons coconut flour
- 2 teaspoon salt

Directions:

1. Chop tuna into tiny pieces.
2. Mash the avocado and combine it with the chopped tuna.
3. Beat the egg into the mixture and add the salt. Stir well.
4. Make small balls and sprinkle them with the coconut flakes and coconut flour.
5. Pour the olive oil in the slow cooker.
6. Add the tuna balls and close the lid.
7. Cook the meal for 2 hours on High.
8. Serve the cooked meal hot!

Baked Mushrooms With Pesto & Ricotta

Ingredients:

- 2 finely chopped cloves of garlic
- 26 grams of freshly grated parmesan cheese
- 2 tablespoons of fresh, chopped parsley
- 35 large chestnut mushrooms
- A 26 0-gram tub of ricotta
- 2 tablespoons of pesto

Directions:

1. Trim the mushroom stems level with the caps.
2. In a small bowl combine the garlic, pesto and ricotta, and spoon into the mushroom heads.

3. Place the mushroom caps in a slow cooker and cook on low for 4-6 hours.
4. In the last half-hour, sprinkle the parmesan cheese over the top of the mushrooms.
5. Serve topped with the fresh parsley.

Beef Stew With Tomatoes

Ingredients:

- 2 c. beef broth
- 2 tbsp. of Chili mix (pre-packaged)
- 2 tbsp. of Worcestershire sauce
- Salt to taste
- 2 cans chili-ready diced tomatoes
- 2 t. hot sauce

Directions:

1. Warm up the slow cooker on the high setting.
2. Add the stewing beef, tomatoes, hot sauce, broth, Worcestershire sauce, chili mix, and salt in the slow cooker.
3. Set the timer for six hours.
4. Break the meat apart and continue cooking for another two hours.
5. Sprinkle with a pinch of salt to taste when ready to serve.

Haloumi, Chorizo And Brussel's Sprout Breakfast Bowl

Ingredients:

- 35 Brussel's sprouts, cut in half
- 2 garlic cloves, crushed
- 4 fresh eggs
- 1 lb haloumi cheese, cut into small pieces
- 2 chorizo sausages, cut into small pieces

Directions:

1. Drizzle some olive oil into the Crock Pot.
2. Add the haloumi, chorizo, Brussel's sprouts, garlic, salt, and pepper to the Crock Pot, stir to combine.

3. Place the lid onto the pot and set the temperature at HIGH.
4. Cook for 2 hours or until the sprouts are cooked.
5. If you wish, you can finish the dish off by quickly sautéing the whole lot in a hot fry pan or skillet until golden and crispy.
6. Serve on 4 plates, with a poached egg on top.
7. Serve while hot!

Zoodle Meatball Soup

Ingredients:

- 4 tsp garlic salt
- 2 tomato, diced
- 2 carrot, chopped
- 2 small onion, diced
- 2 celery ribs, chopped
- 2 medium zucchini, spiralized
- 2 tbsp. olive oil
- 4 2 oz. chicken stock, low-sodium
- 4 tsp sea salt
- 2 tsp oregano
- 2 tsp Italian seasoning
- 4 tsp fresh onion powder
- 4 tbsp. fresh parsley, chopped
- 4 garlic cloves, minced
- 1 cup parmesan cheese, shredded
- 4 lbs. ground beef

Directions:

1. Add beef stock, garlic salt, tomato, carrot, onion, celery, and zucchini into the slow cooker. Stir well.
2. In a large bowl, combine ground beef, pepper, Italian seasoning, oregano, fresh onion powder, sea salt, parsley, egg, garlic, and parmesan cheese.
3. Make45 small meatballs from meat mixture.
4. Heat olive oil in a pan over medium-high heat.
5. Once the oil is hot then add meatballs and cook until lightly brown on all sides.
6. Transfer meatballs to the slow cooker and stir well.
7. Cover and cook on low for 6 hours.
8. Stir well and serve.

Autumn Sweet Chicken

Ingredients:

- 2 boneless and skinless chicken leg
- 2 tablespoons / 28 gr olive oil
- 2 tablespoons / 28 gr ghee
- 2 pinch of fresh onion powder
- 2 dash of fresh lemon juice
- 4 4 cc / 2 fl oz of chicken broth
- 2 pinch of rosemary
- 1 cinnamon stick
- 2 tablespoons / 28 gr of walnuts, roasted
- 2 pinch of ground cinnamon
- 2 pinch of ground nutmeg
- 2 pinch of ground turmeric
- A pinch of salt

Directions:

1. Roast the walnuts in a frying pan. Remove from the stove and set aside to cool

2. Divide in half and use a blender to crumble half of them

3. Mix the Stevia, ground cinnamon, turmeric, nutmeg, and salt in a large bowl. Add the skinless chicken and roll it so it is covered evenly

4. Heat a frying pan and sauté the chicken until golden

5. Dissolve the butter in the same pan on medium heat.

6. Add the onions powder, chopped nuts, fresh lemon juice, and broth, into your Slow Cooker pot with a spoon. Add the spicy chicken and the remaining spice mixture

7. Add by mixing the garlic clove, rosemary and cinnamon stick

8. Cover and cook on LOW for 6-6 ½ hours

Sausage Cauliflower Breakfast Casserole

Ingredients:

- 6 green onions, chopped
- 4 large eggs, beaten
- 1 c. mozzarella cheese, shredded
- 4 tbsp. unsalted butter, melted
- 2 tsps. Salt
- 2 -pound breakfast sausage

Directions:

1. Take the chopped cauliflower at the bottom of the Crockpot. Pour butter and season with salt.
2. Take the sausages and onions on top of the cauliflower bed.
3. Pour over the beaten fresh eggs and top with mozzarella cheese.

4. Cook on low for 4 hours.

Creamy Fresh Eggs

Ingredients:

- 2 teaspoon salt
- 6 eggs, beaten
- 1/2 cup heavy cream
- 2 teaspoon turmeric powder
- 2 teaspoon coriander, ground
- 1 teaspoon ground black pepper
- 2 tablespoon fresh parsley, chopped
- ¾ teaspoon garlic powder
- 1 teaspoon chili flakes
- 2 tablespoon butter
- 4 oz Mozzarella, shredded

Directions:

1. In the mixing bowl, combine the fresh eggs with the cream and the other

ingredients except the butter and the Mozzarella and whisk.

2. Put the butter in the slow cooker.
3. Add the fresh eggs mix, sprinkle the cheese on top, close the lid and cook the casserole for 8 hours on Low. The casserole is cooked, when the egg mixture is set.

Breakfast Meat Bowl

Ingredients:

- 2 garlic clove, chopped
- 2 teaspoon turmeric
- 2 teaspoon paprika
- 4 oz ground chicken
- 4 oz ground beef
- 2 teaspoon tomato puree
- 2 tablespoon butter

Directions:

1. Mix together the ground chicken and ground beef.
2. Sprinkle the meat mixture with the tomato puree and chopped garlic clove.
3. Add turmeric and paprika.
4. Stir the mixture well.

5. Place the butter in the slow cooker and add the ground meat mixture.
6. Close the lid and cook the meal for 4 hours on High.
7. When the meat is cooked, transfer it to serving bowls.
8. Enjoy!
- Nutrition Info: calories 2 46 , fat 6.10 , fiber 0.4, carbs 4 , protein 2 8

Cheddar Spinach Breakfast Quiche

Ingredients:

- 4 cups cheddar cheese
- 2 large bell pepper, finely chopped
- 2 cups mushrooms
- 1/2 tsp baking soda
- 1 cup almond flour
- 2 cup sour cream
- 8 fresh eggs

Directions:

1. Butter or grease your slow cooker.
2. Stir the baking soda in with the almond flour.
3. Whisk the fresh eggs together.
4. Add the sour cream, cheese, bell pepper, and mushroom.

5. Gently fold in the almond and baking powder mixture.
6. Pour everything into the slow cooker.
7. Put the top on the crock pot and adjust the heat setting to high.
8.
9. Cook 2.6 hours remove and cut into 6 pieces. Serve hot and enjoy!

Ginger And Carrot Vichyssoise

Ingredients:

- 2 bay leaf
- 1/2 cup organic orange juice
- 4 cups vegetable or chicken broth
- 1 tsp salt
- 1/2 tsp black pepper
- 1 cup coconut cream, chilled
- Snipped fresh chives
- 1 Tbsp olive oil
- 1 tsp finely minced garlic
- 1/3 Tbsp finely minced ginger root
- 1 white part of leek, washed thoroughly and sliced thinly

- 4 large carrots, peeled and cut into 2 inch thick pieces
- 2 large sweet potato, peeled and sliced in half, then sliced into 2 inch thick pieces

Instructions:

1. Put a large skillet over medium low flame and heat the oil.

2. Sauté the minced garlic, ginger root, and leek for 5 minutes, or until the leeks become tender.

3. Scrape into a 2 quart slow cooker.

4. Put the carrots, sweet potato, bay leaf, orange juice, and broth into the slow cooker.

5. Add the salt and pepper, then stir well. Cover and cook for 6 to 8 hours on low

or until the carrots and sweet potato pieces become tender.

6. Take out the bay leaf and pour the soup into a blender.

7. Puree, then pour into a large soup bowl.

8. Add the chilled coconut cream and stir to combine.

9. Serve warm topped with chives, or cover the container and refrigerate and serve chilled.

Cheesy Sweet Potato And Bacon Soup

Ingredients:

- 4 lb sweet potatoes, peeled and diced
- 4 cups chicken stock
- 4 cups grated sharp cheddar cheese
- 4 tsp fresh thyme or 1/2 tsp dried
- 1/3 cup half and half
- Sea salt
- Freshly ground black pepper
- 4 bacon strips, chopped
- 2 small carrot, diced
- 2 small onion, diced
- 2 celery rib, diced
- 2 large garlic clove, minced

Instructions:

1. Cook the bacon to a crisp in a skillet over medium high flame.

2. Drain on paper towels and set aside. Save 2 tablespoons of grease in the skillet.

3. Using the same skillet, sauté the onion, celery, carrot, and garlic until fresh onion is translucent. Transfer to the slow cooker.

4. Stir in the chicken stock, thyme, and sweet potatoes.

5. Cover and cook for 6 hours on low or for 4 hours on high, or until the sweet potatoes are fork tender.

6. Set heat to high, then mash the mixture using a potato masher.

7. Stir in the half and half and two thirds of the cheddar cheese.

8. Cook for 25 minutes or until the cheese has melted.

9. Season with salt and pepper to taste, then ladle into 6 bowls.

10.   Crumble the bacon and sprinkle over the soup.

11.   Add the remaining cheese on top, then serve.

Beef Vegetable Soup

Ingredients:

- 1 Tbsp dried minced fresh onion
- 1 tsp garlic powder
- 1 tsp kosher salt
- 2 tsp dried Italian seasoning

- 8 ounces frozen mixed vegetables, thawed
- 1 lb beef stew meat
- 2 4 ounces canned stewed tomatoes, undrained
- 1 Tbsp coconut aminos

Instructions:

1. Put the beef in a 4 quart slow cooker and add the canned tomatoes. pour some water into the empty can and pour this into the slow cooker.

2. Add the coconut aminos, salt, garlic powder, Italian seasoning, and dried onion. Add the vegetables and stir to combine.

3. Cover the slow cooker and cook for 8 hours on low, or until the meat can be shredded.

4. Shred the meat and ladle into soup bowls, then serve.

Caribbean Seafood Chowder

Ingredients:

- 1/3 Tbsp grated fresh ginger
- 1/3 Tbsp curry powder
- 1/2 tsp ground cinnamon
- 2 large sweet potato, peeled and diced
- 35 oz canned light coconut milk
- 4 /2 cups seafood stock
- 1/2 lb cod or halibut fillet, rinsed and diced
- Sea salt

- Freshly ground black pepper
- 2 garlic cloves, minced
- 2 small onion, chopped
- 4 Tbsp olive oil
- 2 medium carrot, diced
- 1 red bell pepper, diced
- 1 large Serrano chili or jalapeno, seeded and minced

Instructions:

1. Heat the oil in a skillet over medium high flame.

2. Sauté the onion, carrot, chili, bell pepper, and garlic until fresh onion is translucent.

3. Set heat to low, then add the ginger, cinnamon, and curry powder.

4. Stir for 2 minute, then transfer to the slow cooker.

5. Add the seafood stock, sweet potato, and coconut milk in the slow cooker.

6. Mix well.

7. Cover and cook for 6 hours on low or for 2 hours and 45 minutes on high, or until vegetables are fork tender.

8. Take out a third of the solids using a slotted spoon, then puree in a blender or food processor.

9. Return to the soup and stir.

10. Set slow cooker heat to high, then add the fish fillet and cook for 45 minutes or until fish is cooked through.

11. Season with salt and pepper to taste, then serve piping hot.

Rhode Island Clam Chowder

Ingredients:

- 4 Tbsp snipped fresh dill
- 1 tsp salt
- 2 tsp black pepper
- Cayenne pepper
- 1 lb. flash frozen clam meat or 4 1 ounces canned chopped clams, drained
- 4 slices bacon, sliced into 1 inch pieces
- 1/3 cup chopped sweet onions
- 4 ounces bottled clam juice
- 4 cups sweet potatoes, peeled and diced to 1 inch pieces
- 4 cups chicken broth

Instructions

1. Place a skillet over medium flame and cook the bacon to a crisp.

2. Transfer on paper towels with a slotted spoon and reserve only 1 tablespoon of the bacon fat on the skillet.

3. Sauté the onions in the same skillet until browned, then scrape the onions into a 2 quart slow cooker.

4. Add the bacon, sweet potatoes, chicken broth, clam juice, dill, salt, black pepper, and a dash of cayenne pepper.

5. Stir well. Cover and cook for 6 hours on low.

6. Add the clams and stir to distribute. Cover and cook for an additional half hour. Serve immediately.

Manhattan Clam Chowder

Ingredients:

- 1 green bell pepper, chopped
- 6 oz bottled clam juice
- 2 medium sweet potatoes, scrubbed and diced
- 22 oz canned crushed tomatoes, undrained
- 2 Tbsp chopped fresh parsley
- 1/3 Tbsp fresh thyme or 1/2 tsp dried
- 4 tsp fresh oregano or 1/2 tsp dried
- 4 bay leaves
- Sea salt
- Freshly ground black pepper
- 4 Tbsp olive oil

- 4 pints minced fresh clams
- 2 medium onion, diced
- 4 celery ribs, diced
- 2 large garlic clove, minced
- 2 small carrot, diced

Instructions:

1. Drain the fresh clams, collecting the juice in a bowl. Refrigerate the clams.

2. Place a skillet over medium flame and heat the olive oil. Sauté the onion, carrot, celery, green pepper, and garlic until fresh onion is translucent.

3. Transfer mixture into the slow cooker.

4. Add the sweet potato, tomatoes with juices, parsley, oregano, bay leaves, thyme, clam juice, and juice from fresh clams in the slow cooker.

5. Mix everything well.

6. Cover and cook for 6 hours on low or for 4 hours on high.

7. Set heat to high, then stir in the minced clams.

8. Cook for an additional 25 minutes, or until clams are cooked through.

9. Remove the bay leaf, then season with salt and pepper to taste. Serve at once.

Fresh Salmon Chowder With Sweet Potato

Ingredients:

- 1 lb salmon steaks, cut into 2 inch cubes

- 1/2 tsp dry mustard
- 1/2 tsp dried marjoram leaves
- 1 cup almond or coconut milk
- 2 Tbsp almond or coconut flour
- Salt
- 4 cups fish stock or clam juice, divided
- 2 1/3 cups peeled and cubed sweet potatoes
- 1 cup chopped fresh onion
- White pepper

Instructions:

1. Mix together the sweet potatoes, onion, stock, marjoram, and dry mustard in the slow cooker.

2. Cover and cook for 6 hours on high.

3. Pour the contents into a blender or a food processor and process until

smooth, then pour the chowder back into the slow cooker.

4. Add the salmon and stir, then cover and cook for 10 minutes on high or until the salmon is well done.

5. Combine the milk and flour, then stir this for 2 minutes into the chowder to thicken a bit.

6. Season with salt and white pepper to taste, then serve immediately.

Cold Mint Pea Soup

Ingredients:

- 1 cup sour cream
- 1/2 cup light cream

- Sea salt
- Freshly ground black pepper
- Shredded fresh mint
- 4 Tbsp unsalted butter
- 4 cups chicken stock
- 2 small onion, chopped
- 1/2 lb boiled sweet potatoes, peeled and diced
- 35 oz frozen peas, thawed
- 4 Tbsp chopped fresh mint
- 4 Tbsp chopped fresh parsley

Instructions:

1. Place a skillet over medium high flame and heat the butter. Sauté the fresh onion until translucent, then pour contents into the slow cooker.

2. Add the potatoes, peas, parsley, mint, and chicken stock. Stir gently.

3. Cover and cook for 6 hours on low or for 2 hours and45 minutes on high.

4. Set heat to high, then stir in the light cream. Cook for 35 minutes.

5. Turn off the heat, then let stand for half an hour. Puree using a food processor or immersion blender.

6. Season with salt and pepper to taste, then refrigerate for half an hour or until chilled.

7. Ladle into 6 soup bowls, then top with sour cream and shredded fresh mint. Serve at once.

Turkey And Broccoli Chili

Ingredients:

- 2 red bell pepper, seeded and diced
- 2 tsp ground cumin
- 1 tsp dried Italian seasoning
- 1/2 tsp kosher salt
- 1/2 tsp ground black pepper
- 2 cup chicken broth
- Optional: sour cream
- 1/3 lb broccoli florets, roughly chopped
- 1 lb ground turkey
- 1 onion, diced
- 2 cloves garlic, diced
- 1 Tbsp chili powder

124

Instructions:

1. Place a skillet over medium flame and sauté the turkey, onion, and garlic until the turkey is completely browned. Crumble it up with a fork.

2. Using a slotted spoon, transfer the mixture into the slow cooker.

3. Add the bell pepper, chili powder, cumin, Italian seasoning, and broth.

4. Stir well, cover, and cook for 8 hours on low.

5. Season with salt and pepper, ladle into soup bowls, and serve with a dollop of sour cream on top, if desired.

Szechwan Hot And Sour Soup

Makes: 6 servings

Ingredients:

- 4 Tbsp coconut aminos
- 1/3 Tbsp Asian sesame oil
- 4 Tbsp almond flour
- 4 small fresh eggs
- 1/2 tsp freshly ground black pepper
- 4 scallions, trimmed and sliced thinly
- 10 large dried shiitake mushrooms
- 1/2 lb boneless pork loin, fat trimmed
- 1/3 cup boiling water
- 4 1 cups chicken stock
- 4 Tbsp rice wine vinegar

Instructions:

1. Soak the mushrooms in the boiled water for 35 minutes. Set aside.

2. Slice the pork thinly into ribbons, then place inside the slow cooker.

3. Strain the mushrooms, saving the liquid in a bowl.

4. Remove the stems, then slice the caps thinly.

5. Transfer to the slow cooker.

6. Add the stock, vinegar, coconut aminos, pepper, and sesame oil. Mix everything well.

7. Cover and cook for 6 hours on low or for 4 hours on high, or until pork is cooked through.

8. Set heat to high.

9. In a bowl, combine 4 tablespoons cold water with the almond flour, then stir into the soup. Cook for 35 minutes, or until bubbly.

10.   Beat the fresh eggs in a bowl, then slowly pour into the soup. Cover and cook for 35 minutes, or until simmering.

11.   Season with salt and pepper to taste, then ladle into 6 bowls. Top with sliced scallions, then serve.

Chunky Meaty Chili

Ingredients:

- 8 ounces chopped broccoli florets
- 1/2 cup chopped sweet onions
- 2 Tbsp chili powder
- 1/2 tsp garlic powder
- 1 tsp salt, divided
- 1 tsp ground cumin
- 2 /35 tsp ground cinnamon
- Optional: 1/2 cup shredded cheddar cheese
- 1 lb boneless beef chuck roast (excess fat trimmed off), sliced into 1/3 inch pieces
- 1 lb pork tenderloin, sliced into 1/3 inch pieces

- 1 tablespoon olive oil
- 1/9 cup almond flour
- 35 ounces canned diced tomatoes and green chilies, with juices

Instructions:

1. Combine the beef and pork in a large mixing bowl.

2. Sprinkle the flour on top and mix toss to coat the pieces in the flour.

3. Place a large skillet over medium flame and heat the olive oil.

4. Cook the meat until browned all over, then transfer the meat into a 4 quart slow cooker using a slotted spoon.

5. Add the tomatoes, broccoli, onions, chili powder, garlic powder, salt, cumin, and cinnamon into the slow cooker with the meats. Stir well.

6.   Cover and cook for 6 to 6 hours on low, or until the meats are well done and tender.

7. Serve in soup bowls and top with shredded cheddar cheese, if desired.

Sweet Roots And Steak Chili

Ingredients:

4 Tbsp olive oil

4 lb top sirloin steak, cubed

1/3 Tbsp ground cumin

2 Tbsp chili powder

Chopped green fresh onion

- 4 carrots, peeled and cubed
- 4 sweet potatoes, peeled and cubed
- 2 red bell pepper, chopped
- 35 oz canned diced tomatoes with green chilies
- 2 medium onion, chopped
- 4 garlic cloves, crushed
- 35 oz beef broth

Instructions:

1. Heat the olive oil in a skillet over medium-high flame.

2. Brown the cubed steak, then drain and set aside.

3. Place the carrots, sweet potatoes, bell pepper, tomatoes with green chilies, onion, garlic, and broth into the slow cooker.

4. Stir in the chili powder and cumin.

134

5. Add the steak into the slow cooker, then cover and cook for 8 hours on low.

6. Ladle into 6 bowls, then sprinkle green onions and serve immediately.

Chili Verde

Ingredients:

- 1 green bell pepper, chopped
- 4 oz Monterrey Jack cheese
- 1/2 cup chopped cilantro
- 1 tsp ground cumin
- 1 tsp dried oregano
- Sea salt
- Black pepper
- 6 corn tortillas, sliced into wedges

- 1 cup cooked beans
- 1 lb boneless, skinless chicken breast
- 1/3 cup salsa Verde
- 2 celery rib, chopped
- 2 clove garlic, minced
- 2 small onion, chopped

Instructions:

1. Combine the chicken, celery, garlic, onion, bell pepper, and salsa Verde in the slow cooker.

2. Season with cumin, oregano, and salt and pepper to taste.

3. Cover and cook for 6 hours on low.

4. Stir in the beans and use a fork to break up the chicken.

5. Cook for 2 hour on low.

6. Preheat the oven to 450degrees F. Coat a baking sheet with non-stick cooking spray.

7. Arrange the corn tortillas on the prepared baking sheet and bake for 2 minutes to a crisp.

8. Remove the chili from the heat and sprinkle the cheese on top.

9. Stir until melted, then top with cilantro. Ladle into soup bowls and serve with the corn tortillas.

Parsnip And Pumpkin Soup

Ingredients:

- 2 Tbsp coconut oil
- 1 Tbsp ginger, minced
- 1/2 tsp cilantro
- 1/2 tsp cumin
- 1/2 tsp salt
- 2 cup vegetable stock
- 1 pumpkin, peeled and cubed
- 2 small onion, chopped
- 2 parsnip, diced
- 1 clove garlic, minced
- Optional: 1 cup ham and/or 2 Tbsp chopped chives

Instructions:

1. Combine the parsnip and pumpkin in the slow cooker.

2. Place a saucepan over medium flame and heat the olive oil.

3. Sauté the onion, garlic, ginger, cilantro, salt, and cumin until fragrant.

4. Pour in the vegetable stock.

5. Let boil then pour into the slow cooker.

6. Season with more salt, if needed. Cover and cook for 6 hours on low.

7. Ladle into soup bowls and top with ham and chives.

Ham And Potato Chowder

Ingredients:

- 4 cup cubed ham steak
- 6 cups diced potato
- 4 1 cups chicken broth
- 4 cups heavy cream
- 4 cups chopped fresh onion
- 4 cloves garlic, minced
- 2 tsp salt
- Black pepper
- 2 Tbsp chopped green fresh onion

Instructions:

1. Combine the ham, potato, broth, onion, and garlic in the slow cooker.

2. Cover and cook for 6 hours on low.

3. Stir in the heavy cream and cook for an additional 2 hour on low.

4. Ladle into soup bowls and top with green onion. Serve immediately.

Spicy Cauliflower Soup

Ingredients:

- 4 Tbsp tomato paste
- 4 jalapeno peppers, diced

- 2 cloves garlic, minced
- 4 tsp oregano
- 4 tsp ground cumin
- Salt
- Black pepper
- 2 large cauliflower head, stem cut off, florets chopped
- 2 red bell peppers, diced
- 2 green bell pepper, diced
- 2 large onion, diced
- 2 cups tomato sauce
- 2 cup chicken stock

Instructions:

1. Combine the tomato paste, tomato sauce, and chicken stock in the slow cooker.

2. Stir in the oregano and cumin, then the onion, bell peppers and jalapeno peppers.

3. Stir in the cauliflower to coat thoroughly. Add just enough water to cover the ingredients.

4. Cover the slow cooker and cook for 6 hours on low.

5. Mash the ingredients with a potato masher, or pour into a food processor and puree.

6. Season to taste with salt and pepper. Serve chilled or warm.

Spicy And Sour Shrimp Soup

Ingredients:

- 4 Tbsp rice wine vinegar
- 4 Tbsp coconut aminos
- 1/2 tsp white pepper
- 1/2 tsp red pepper flakes
- 1 lb shrimp, peeled and deveined
- 2 eggs, whisked
- 6 cups chicken broth
- 35 oz bamboo shoots
- 2   carrot, cut into matchstick thin strips
- 4 oz water chestnuts, drained
- 1 cup sliced mushrooms

Instructions:

1. Pour the chicken broth, bamboo shoots, carrot, chestnuts, mushroom, vinegar, coconut aminos, white pepper, and red pepper flakes in the slow cooker.

2. Cover and cook for 8 hours on low or for 4 hours on high.

3. Add the shrimp, cover and cook for 2 hour on low.

4. Gradually pour the whisked egg into the soup as you twirl the surface of the soup with a fork to distribute the egg.

5. Ladle into soup bowls and serve immediately.

Chicken Dumpling Soup

Ingredients:

- 1/2 cup milk
- 2 small onion, sliced
- 1 Tbsp coriander
- Salt
- Black pepper
- 1 lb skinless chicken breast, sliced into chunks
- 2 cup chicken broth
- 6 oz mixed vegetables (such as corn kernels, peas, and diced carrots)
- 1 cup rice or almond flour

Instructions:

1. Combine the onion, mixed vegetables, and cubed chicken in the slow cooker.

2. Pour the broth all over and stir to mix. Cover and cook for 6 hours on low.

3. Combine the milk and flour in a small bowl, then spoon the mixture gradually into the slow cooker and stir until the soup slightly thickens.

4. Cook for an additional hour on low.

5. Season to taste with salt and pepper.

6. Sprinkle coriander on top and serve piping hot.

Split Pea Soup

Ingredients:

- 2 bay leaf
- 1/2 cup chopped fresh parsley
- 2 cup water
- 1 Tbsp dried thyme
- 1 Tbsp olive oil
- Salt
- Black pepper
- 1 lb split green peas
- 2 cups vegetable broth
- 1 cup chopped baby carrots
- 2 celery stalks, chopped
- 2 small onion, chopped
- 2 clove garlic, minced

Instructions:

1. Soak the peas in a bowl of water for 4 hours, then drain thoroughly and pour into the slow cooker.

2. Stir the carrots, celery, garlic, onion, parsley, thyme and bay leaf into the slow cooker and season with salt and pepper.

3. Pour the stock all over the ingredients and stir to combine.

4. Cover and cook for 8 hours on low, or until the peas are fork tender. Serve hot.

Hungarian Soup

Ingredients:

- 2 Tbsp chopped fresh dill
- 1 Tbsp paprika
- 1 Tbsp olive oil
- 1 tsp celery seeds
- 1/2 tsp salt
- 1/9 tsp ground nutmeg
- Black pepper
- 2 lb russet potatoes, scrubbed and cubed
- 2 cups vegetable broth, unsalted
- 1 cup skimmed milk
- 2 small onion, minced
- 1/2 cup corn kernels

Instructions:

1. Combine the potatoes, paprika, celery seeds, and vegetable broth in the slow cooker. Mix well.

2. Place a skillet over medium flame and heat the olive oil.

3. Sauté the fresh onion until tender then scrape into the slow cooker.

4. Cover the slow cooker and cook for 4 hours on low, or until potatoes are very tender.

5. Break up the potatoes using a fork, then stir in the dill, nutmeg, salt and pepper.

6. Pour in the milk and stir to combine.

7. Cook for additional 210 minutes on low.

8. Adjust seasoning, if needed. Ladle into soup bowls and serve piping hot.

Hungarian Goulash

Ingredients:

- 1 Tbsp Worcestershire sauce (gluten free) or coconut aminos
- 1 tsp hot ground mustard powder
- 1/2 cup tomato paste
- 2 tsp paprika
- 2 medium size sweet potatoes, peeled and sliced into 4 inch pieces
- 2 tbsp almond flour
- Salt
- Freshly ground black pepper
- Sour coconut or almond cream
- 1 teaspoon olive oil

- 4 lbs boneless chuck roast, sliced into 4 inch pieces
- 1/2 tsp coarse salt
- 1/2 tsp cracked black pepper
- 1/9 cup molasses
- 1/9 cup fresh lime juice
- 1/2 tsp garlic powder

Instructions:

1. Place a skillet over medium flame and heat the olive oil.

2. Season the meat with salt and pepper, then brown it in the skillet.

3. Using a slotted spoon, put the browned meat into a 4 quart slow cooker.

4. Sprinkle the onions on top of the meat.

5. In a bowl, combine the molasses, garlic powder, mustard powder, lime juice,

Worcestershire sauce or coconut aminos, tomato paste, and paprika.

6. Pour the mixture all over the meat and onions.

7. Cover the slow cooker and cook for 6 hours on low.

8. Add the sweet potatoes and cook for an additional hour, or until the sweet potatoes become fork tender.

9. Using a slotted spoon, put the meat, sweet potatoes, and onions into a large mixing bowl and pour about 1/3 of the cooking liquid into a saucepan.

10.   Place the saucepan over medium flame.

11.   Put the almond flour into a small mixing bowl and beat in the remaining cooking liquid from the slow cooker to create a paste.

12.   Put the meat, sweet potatoes, and onions back into the slow cooker.

13.   Cover and set the slow cooker to warm.

14.   Add the almond flour mixture into the saucepan and mix until the liquids start to thicken. Season to taste with salt and pepper.

15.   Arrange the meat, sweet potatoes, and onions on a serving platter, then pour the sauce on top and serve with the sour cream.

Herbed Pot Roast

Ingredients:

- 1/2 cup chopped fresh rosemary or 2 Tbsp dried
- 2 Tbsp chopped fresh thyme or 2 tsp dried
- 4 Tbsp almond flour
- Sea salt
- Freshly ground black pepper
- 4 lb boneless chuck or rump roast
- 2 large sweet onions
- 1/2 cup olive oil
- 6 garlic cloves, minced
- 4 cups beef stock
- 4 carrots, sliced
- 4 Tbsp chopped fresh parsley

Instructions:

1. Preheat the broiler in the oven. Line a broiler pan with aluminum foil.

2. Broil the roast for 10 minutes per side.

3. Place the roast into the slow cooker together with the juices in the pan.

4. Place a skillet over medium high flame and heat the oil.

5. Sauté the fresh onion and garlic until fresh onion is translucent.

6. Transfer to the slow cooker.

7. Add the carrots, rosemary, celery, and stock into the slow cooker. Mix the ingredients well.

8. Cover and cook for 35 hours on low or for 6 hours on high, or until the beef is extremely tender.

9. Turn off the heat and let stand for45 minutes to an hour.

10. Remove the fat that accumulates at the top of the mixture.

11. Set heat to high.

12. Combine the almond flour with 4 tablespoons of cold water in bowl, then stir the mixture into the slow cooker.

13. Cover and cook for 25 minutes, or until sauce is thickened.

14. Season with salt and pepper to taste, then serve at once.

Red Cooked Beef

Ingredients:

- 2 scallions, sliced in half lengthwise and cut into three pieces
- 1/2 cup coconut aminos
- 1/2 tsp finely minced garlic
- 1/2 Tbsp raw honey or maple syrup

- 1/3 cup water
- 2 lbs skirt steak
- 4 Tbsp olive oil
- 1/3 inch ginger root, peeled and sliced thinly

Instructions:

1. Place a skillet over medium high flame and heat the oil.

2. Sear the steak for 35 seconds per side, then transfer immediately into a 2 quart slow cooker.

3. Put the ginger root slices and scallions on top of the meat.

4. In a small bowl, beat together the coconut aminos, raw honey or maple syrup, and garlic.

5. Gradually stir in the water. Pour the mixture all over the meat.

6. Cover the slow cooker and cook for 4 hours on low, or until the meat is medium-rare.

7. Slice the steak and serve with the sauce.

Moroccan Lamb Stew

Ingredients:

- 4 carrots, sliced thickly
- 6 Tbsp balsamic vinegar
- 2 cup pimiento stuffed green olives
- 1 lb dried apricots, sliced
- 1 cup raw honey or high quality maple syrup
- 4 Tbsp chopped fresh oregano or 2 Tbsp dried
- 4 tsp ground cumin
- 4 Tbsp almond flour
- Sea salt
- Freshly ground black pepper
- 4 lb boneless lamb shoulder, cubed
- 4 Tbsp olive oil

- 6 garlic cloves, minced
- 2 large sweet onions, diced
- 2 small jalapeno or Serrano chili, seeded and minced
- 4 cups dry red wine
- 4 cups beef stock
- 4 parsnips, sliced thickly

Instructions:

1. Preheat the broiler. Line a broiler pan using aluminum foil.

2. Broil the lamb until browned, then transfer to the slow cooker with the juices in the pan.

3. Place a skillet over medium high flame and heat the oil.

4. Sauté the onion, garlic, and chili until fresh onion is translucent.

5. Transfer mixture into the slow cooker.

6. Add the stock, wine, vinegar, parsnips, carrots, olives, dried apricots, honey or maple syrup, cumin, and oregano. Mix well.

7. Cover and cook for 35 hours on low or for 6 hours on high, or until lamb is extremely tender.

8. Combine the almond flour with 4 tablespoons of cold water in a bowl.

9. Increase heat to high and stir the mixture into the slow cooker.

10.   Cover and cook for 25 minutes, or until sauce has thickened.

11.   Season with salt and pepper to taste, then serve.

Fresh Lemon And Artichoke Veal Stew

Ingredients:

- 1 cup chopped sweet onions
- 1/2 tsp crushed red pepper flakes
- 2 tsp freshly grated fresh lemon peel
- 85 ounces canned whole artichokes, rinsed, drained, and cut into quarters
- 4 Tbsp white wine
- 1/3 cup chicken broth
- 1/9 cup fresh fresh lemon juice
- 2 large egg
- 1/2 cup snipped fresh flat leaf parsley, divided
- 1 lb wide gluten-free egg noodles
- 1/2 cup almond flour

172

- 1/3 tsp salt, divided
- 1/2 tsp black pepper, divided
- 4 lbs veal stew meat, sliced into 2 inch cubes
- 4 Tbsp olive oil, divided
- 2 tsp finely minced garlic

Instructions:

1. Combine the almond flour, half the salt, and half the pepper in a large resealable plastic back.

2. Put the veal into the bag and shake to coat. Put the coated pieces on a plate.

3. Place a skillet over medium flame and heat half of the olive oil.

4. Brown the veal for about half a minute per side, then transfer the pieces into a 4 quart slow cooker.

5. Wipe the skillet clean and heat the remaining oil in it.

6. Sauté the onions, garlic, fresh lemon peel, crushed red pepper, and artichokes.

7. Season with the remaining salt and pepper.

8. Cook until the vegetables are all tender.

9. Pour the broth and fresh lemon juice into the skillet and increase the heat to high.

10. Bring to a boil for about a minute, then pour the mixture into the slow cooker and stir to combine the ingredients well.

11. Cover the slow cooker and cook for 4 hours on low.

12. Using a slotted spoon take the veal and artichokes out of the slow cooker and place them in a bowl.

13.   Use aluminum foil to cover the bowl and keep the contents warm.

14.   In a bowl, beat together the fresh eggs and 1/3 of the parsley.

15.   Season with a bit of salt. Pour the mixture into the slow cooker and cover.

16.   Cook for 8 minutes on high, then put the veal and artichokes back into the slow cooker. Stir well.

17.   Cover and cook for an additional 35 minutes on high.

18.   Cook the noodles based on the manufacturer's instructions, then drain and divide between three serving plates.

19.   Top the noodles with the veal and artichoke sauce and garnish with the remaining parsley.

Veal Paprikash

Ingredients:

- 1/2 cup vegetable oil
- 4 lb veal stew meat
- 6 Tbsp paprika
- 2 large onions, diced
- 6 garlic cloves, minced
- 45 oz canned diced tomatoes, undrained

Instructions:

1. Preheat the broiler.

2. Line a broiler pan using aluminum foil. Broil the meat until browned, about 4 minutes per side.

3. Place into the slow cooker with juices from the pan.

4. Heat half the vegetable oil in a skillet over medium high flame.

5. Sauté the fresh onion and garlic until fresh onion is translucent.

6. Reduce to low flame and add the paprika. Sauté for 2 minute, then transfer mixture into the slow cooker.

7. Add the wine, stock, thyme, and tomatoes into the slow cooker.

8. Cover and cook for 8 hours on low or for 4 hours on high, or until the meat is extra tender.

9. Set heat to high.

10. Combine the almond flour with 4 tablespoons of cold water.

11. Stir mixture into the slow cooker.

12. Cover and cook for 25 minutes, or until thickened.

13. Add the cashew sour cream and cook for 4 minutes. Do not bring to a boil.

14. Season with salt and pepper to taste, then serve.

Cape Malay Lamb Curry

Ingredients:

- 1 tsp peeled and grated ginger root

- 1/2 tsp turmeric
- 1/9 cup fresh fresh lemon juice
- 1 Tbsp tamarind syrup
- 1/2 tsp salt
- 2 Tbsp coconut cream
- 1 cup water
- 4 Tbsp olive oil, divided
- 4 cups thinly sliced sweet onions
- 1 Tbsp finely minced garlic
- 2 lb boneless leg of lamb (all fat trimmed), sliced into 4 inch pieces
- 1/9 tsp salt
- 1 Tbsp red curry paste
- 2 piece Thai herb paste

Instructions:

1. Heat a tablespoon of olive oil in a large skillet over medium flame.

2. Sauté the onions for 4 minutes, then add the minced garlic and sauté for an additional 2 minutes.

3. Scrape the mixture into a 4 quart slow cooker.

4. Heat a tablespoon of oil in the same skillet. Season the lamb with salt, then brown the pieces for 2 minutes over medium flame.

5. Use a slotted spoon to transfer the browned lamb into the slow cooker.

6. In a mixing bowl, stir together the red curry paste, turmeric, herb paste, ginger root, fresh lemon juice, turmeric, tamarind syrup, coconut cream, salt, and water.

7. Pour the mixture into the slow cooker and stir to coat the lamb pieces.

8. Cover the slow cooker and cook for 4 hours on low, or until the lamb is tender

and cooked through. Serve with a plate of hot cauliflower rice.

Greek Beef Stew

Ingredients:

- 4 Tbsp raw honey or high quality maple syrup
- 2 lbs frozen pearl onions, thawed
- 1 cup dried currants
- 4 Tbsp almond flour
- Sea salt
- Freshly ground black pepper
- 4 Tbsp olive oil
- 4 lb stewing beef, fat trimmed
- 6 garlic cloves, minced
- 2 large onions, diced
- 2 tsp ground coriander
- 4 Tbsp chopped fresh oregano or 4 tsp dried

- 2 tsp ground cinnamon
- 2 juice oranges, rinsed thoroughly
- **45**   oz   canned   diced   tomatoes, undrained
- 2 cups beef stock
- 2 cup dry red wine
- 4 Tbsp balsamic vinegar

Instructions:

1. Preheat the broiler.

2. Line a broiler pan using aluminum foil.

3. Broil the beef until browned, about 10 minutes per side.

4. Place beef and juices in the pan into the slow cooker.

5. Heat the oil over medium high flame in a skillet.

6. Sauté the fresh onion and garlic until onions are translucent.

7. Set heat to low and add the cinnamon, coriander, and oregano.

8. Sauté for 2 minute, then transfer everything into the slow cooker.

9. Grate the zest from the oranges and extract the juice.

10.   Add zest and juice to the slow cooker.

11.   Add the tomatoes, wine, stock, honey or maple syrup, vinegar, currants, and pearl onions into the slow cooker. Mix well.

12.   Cover and cook for 35 hours on low or for 6 hours on high, or until the beef is extra tender.

13.   Set heat to high.

14. Combine the almond flour with 4 tablespoons of cold water in a bowl, then stir into the slow cooker.

15. Cover and cook for 25 minutes, or until simmering and thickened.

16. Season with salt and pepper to taste, then serve.

Cherry Pork Stew

Ingredients:

1/3 cup chopped onions

25 ounces canned sugar-free cherry pie filling, divided (gluten free, Paleo)

1 tsp salt

4 Tbsp fresh lemon juice

2 /35 tsp ground nutmeg

- 1/2 tsp crushed red pepper flakes
- 8 ounces chopped broccoli florets
- Salt
- Freshly ground black pepper
- 1/9 cup almond flour
- 1 Tbsp fresh lemon and herb seasoning
- 2 1/2 lbs pork loin roast, sliced into 2 inch cubes
- 2 Tbsp coconut oil or ghee, divided

Instructions:

1. Combine the almond flour and fresh lemon and herb seasoning in a resealable plastic bag.

2. Put the pork into the bag and seal tightly.

3. Shake to coat the pork in the mixture and then transfer the pieces onto a plate.

4. Heat a tablespoon of coconut oil or ghee in a skillet over medium heat.

5. Brown the pork pieces for 4 minutes, then transfer them into a 2 quart slow cooker.

6. Sprinkle the remaining flour and seasoning mixture over the pork in the slow cooker.

7. Heat the remaining oil or ghee in the skillet over medium flame and sauté the onions for 4 minutes, then transfer into the slow cooker.

8. Stir half of the cherry pie filling and all of the fresh lemon juice, nutmeg, red pepper flakes, and salt in the slow cooker. Top the mixture with the remaining cherry pie filling. Cover the slow cooker and cook for 4 hours on low.

9. Add the broccoli florets and stir. Cover and cook for an additional45 minutes.

Season with salt and pepper and serve warm.

Italian Braised Ham

Ingredients:

2 cup dry red wine

2 Tbsp chopped fresh oregano or 2 tsp dried

4 Tbsp chopped fresh parsley

2 Tbsp chopped fresh basil or 2 tsp dried

2 bay leaves

Sea salt

Freshly ground black pepper

4 Tbsp olive oil

6 garlic cloves, minced

4 large onions, sliced thinly

2 green bell pepper, seeded and sliced thinly

- 4 lb baked ham, sliced thickly
- 45 oz canned crushed tomatoes in tomato puree

Instructions:

1. Heat the oil over medium high flame in a skillet.

2. Sauté the onion, bell pepper, and garlic until fresh onion is translucent.

3. Transfer to the slow cooker.

4. Place the ham on top of the fresh onion mixture, then add the wine, tomatoes, parsley, basil, oregano, and bay leaves.

5. Cover and cook for 8 hours on low or for 4-4 ½ hours on high.

6. Take the bay leaves out, then season with salt and pepper to taste. Serve warm.

Indochina Pineapple Pork Stew

Ingredients:

- 2 lb pork loin roast, sliced into 2 inch pieces
- Salt
- Freshly ground black pepper
- 1 Tbsp olive oil
- 2 cup chopped fresh onion
- 2 Tbsp of finely minced garlic
- 2 cup fresh pineapple
- 85 ounces canned petite-diced tomatoes, drained
- 1 cup coconut cream

- 1/2 cup pineapple juice
- 1/9 cup tamarind syrup
- 1 Tbsp chili garlic paste
- 1/9 cup sweet chili sauce, gluten-free
- 1/9 cup teriyaki sauce, gluten-free
- 2 Tbsp coconut aminos
- 2 Tbsp apple cider vinegar
- 4 Tbsp raw honey
- 2 Tbsp almond butter
- 1/2 cup almond flour
- 2 Tbsp ghee

Instructions:

1. Make the Indochina sauce 2 weeks before preparing the dish.

2. In a blender or food processor, combine the coconut cream, pineapple juice, sweet chili sauce, and tamarind syrup. Pulse until smooth.

3. Add the teriyaki sauce, coconut aminos, honey, vinegar, and chili garlic paste.

4. Pulse again until smooth.

5. Add the almond butter and blend until smooth.

6. Scrape the sauce into a tightly sealed container and refrigerate.

7. Put the almond flour in a resealable plastic bag. Add the pork and seal shut.

8. Shake to coat the pork in the flour, then transfer the pork to a plate.

9. Season to taste with salt and pepper.

10. Place a skillet over medium flame and heat the oil.

11. Brown the pork for 4 minutes, then transfer into a 4 quart slow cooker.

12. Use the same skillet to saute the fresh onion and garlic for 2 minutes.

13.   Transfer the fresh onion and garlic to the slow cooker.

14.   Add the tomatoes, pineapple, and about 1 cup of the Indochina sauce into the slow cooker.

15.   Stir well, then cover and cook for 4 hours on low or until the pork is well done. Serve with warm cauliflower rice.

Simple Cabbage And Beef

Ingredients:

4 cups water

1 bay leaf

2 clove garlic

1 tsp brown sugar

1 tsp salt

1 lb potatoes, scrubbed and halved

1 small green cabbage, sliced into wedges

4 lbs corned beef brisket

2 medium carrot, sliced into cubes

Instructions:

1. Combine the carrots, potatoes, bay leaf and garlic in the slow cooker then add the beef on top.

2. Sprinkle the salt and sugar all over the beef then add water.

3. Cover the slow cooker and cook for 8 hours on low.

4. Stir in the cabbage and cook for an additional 2 hour on low.

5. Turn off the heat and let stand to cool for about 10 minutes then remove the bay leaf. Spoon onto plates and serve piping hot.

Pork Tenderloin With Sour Cream

Ingredients:

- 2 medium onion, quartered
- 1/2 cup fresh cilantro
- 2 Tbsp olive oil
- 1 tsp salt
- 1 tsp black pepper
- 1 tsp dried oregano
- 1 tsp ground cumin
- Non-stick cooking spray
- 2 lb pork tenderloin
- 1 cup chicken broth
- 2 red bell pepper, diced
- 4 cloves garlic, minced
- 1 lb fresh tomatillos, sliced in half

- 1 cup sour cream, preferably low fat

Instructions:

1. Broil the tomatillos in the oven for 6 minutes per side.

2. Scrape into a food processor and puree. Set aside.

3. Combine the salt, black pepper, oregano, and cumin.

4. Massage the mixture all over the pork tenderloin.

5. Place a skillet over medium flame and coat with non-stick cooking spray.

6. Sear the meat all over for about 8 minutes then transfer into the slow cooker.

7. Pour the chicken broth and spoon the tomatillo puree into the slow cooker.

8. Add the fresh onion and garlic, and mix well to coat the meat.

9. Season with more salt and black pepper.

10. Cover and cook on low for 6-6 ½ hours.

11. Remove the pork tenderloin from the slow cooker and shred.

12. Pour the sauce all over and serve with a dollop of sour cream.

Zucchini Sausage Breakfast "Bake"

Ingredients:

8 ounces cream cheese

35 large fresh eggs

2 small zucchinis, grated and excess water squeezed

4 cloves of garlic, minced

2 cup cheese, shredded

2 -pound Italian sausages, chopped

1 cup coconut flour

2 teaspoons baking powder

2 teaspoon salt

1 teaspoon pepper

Directions:

Mix all fixings in a bowl. Set in the slow cooker; cook within 4 hours on high or on low for 4 hours.

Nutrition:

Calories: 4 44 Carbohydrates: 6.4 g

Protein: 22 g Fat: 28 g

Sugar: 0.4g

Sodium: 8 4 6mg

Fiber: 4g

Lightning Source UK Ltd.
Milton Keynes UK
UKHW020643270922
409514UK00009B/458